MY AUTISTIC HEART

PAULA NASH

Copyright - **Paula Nash 2022**

Facebook page - **My Autistic Heart**

This book has been created solely from **the use of audio and video transcription materials.** It has been created in my own words, opinion, and the truth as i know it. It can not be reproduced in any manner whatsoever without written permission. To order copies please contact me directly at *paulanash0@gmail.com*

Thank you for taking the time to enter my world. I genuinely appreciate it.

DEDICATION

To God my Creator to you i give my gratitude as it is through your will that this book has been created. I am merely an example.

The hand of God is everpresent and omnipotent and in my life there have been never ending miracles that have come through people, events and divinely orchestrated moments.

That is a story for my next book i am sure.

TABLE OF CONTENTS

PREFACE

I have been divinely guided to write this book. This book is for everyone, whether you are on the Autism Spectrum or not, im wanting to express my heart through the lens of my experiences and how i perceive the world. This is why it is only transcribed directly from a series of audios and videos that i have recorded over a number of years. I expressly feel that it will invite you the reader on a journey into your heart, where you can experience my world for yourself.

I feel that from here you can take from it what you will and i sincerely hope that within the content you will find some inspiration.

Heart to Heart
Paula

ACKNOWLEDGEMENT

To the Earth Angels in human form who have supported me on this journey

I thank you sincerely for standing with me even when in darkness, in suffering, and in hard times. I am Grateful.

Also thank you to those who did not support me and who put me in darkness, in suffering, and in hard times. It was in those times God lifted me, Empowered me, opened my heart, and helped me to survive.

CHAPTER ONE

MY AUTISTIC HEART

I was always sensitive, always empathetic, always feeling the pain of the world. Even from a young age, when I started watching on TV the famine that was going on in Ethiopia, I think it was at the time of Live Aid (Bob Geldof). My heart used to break and I used to be really shocked at what was going on and how it could even be. I think I was only about 5 or 6 at the time. So that was the pain cutting through my whole life. I've always had that sensitivity and I can't comprehend how people can allow other people to suffer in that way; why there can be war and there isn't peace. So, this was the pain that has followed me all through my life. I hope that in a way, I can make some sort of humanitarian difference as time goes on. I'm not sure yet in what way but it's really around ending of suffering and the birth of peace. It's ascension of human consciousness.

That was how my childhood was. I was very much feeling a lot, feeling the pain of the world. So when people say that Autistic people don't have feelings or emotions or whatever, that's just a myth. Every Autistic person I ever met feels so deeply, it's just hard to express, we may express a little differently and the process can be slower with emotions. Something might happen and it will take me some days to actually dig in to feel the emotions. That's learning for us. So although it's there, all the cells in the body in charge of emotions, just that sometimes, we don't know how to express, sometimes, it can take time.

So now, I sit into the body and really try and examine what's going on with the emotion. That's learning. I think it's learning for all of us. For people who are looking from the outside, who are not Autistic, it's really important, it's like everything. We just have a different way, we're just different. People need to take that on board as well at this point. I'm sure there are new studies being done as many of us in the Autistic community are getting involved in the main stream education, health and public service fields. There's a lot of

Autistic people starting to stand and speak for themselves and can explain how it is for them.

There's a vein that runs through all of us in the Autistic community. Definitely, it's similar yet we are very different. It's very individual. I might be telling you something of how it is for me and somebody else will not have that experience.

There's still a lot of work to be done in this area. There are many undiagnosed Autistics as well and people who may not want a diagnosis or whatever. I think it's a signpost. It's a signpost for me to understand my moods, my body, things I liked and things I didn't like. When I was diagnosed first. I had to go back to my feelings, to things I had done in my life. Did I really like to do that? Was that me? Was that something I really liked or was I just playing along? Was I trying to be somebody else or could I have been a chameleon?

So I was like okay, I like this. I studied nursing. Did I want to be a nurse? What did I want to be? I'm just going back into healing and discovering okay, I like this, I don't like this and so on. I discovered the real core of who I am. And that was an awakening and healing and devastation and joy. It's so mixed.

35 years in the dark, feeling lost Who am I? I feel different, just going along with life, trying to do whatever anyone else did, finding it hard to keep to team work, mortgage difficulties, bringing up my children. It wasn't easy. I know it's not easy for anybody. But definitely, it was challenging at all levels, a lot depression, anxiety, panic attacks, sadness, a lot of masking, using alcohol, using cigarettes just to dumb down pain.

At this age, a lot of that pain and depression shifted immediately because you kinda go, "Oh... this is what it is..." and "Oh my God, I don't want to be like this..." Then, eventually I gave in to acceptance. But it took a lot of years to really come to this. Definitely, I like myself a lot. And I even love myself probably now. I'm really kind to me. That's where it begins because I know I'll be kind to other people and less judgmental. We're all in a battle whether it's an Autistic person or not an Autistic person, there's a different kind of battle going on.

As we are here, we are different, going through illusions, going back to source.

But it's revealing, revealing different parts of who we are, different part of our personalities, different aspects of myself, of learned behaviours, of sabotaging behaviours, the old feeling of not being good enough, walking through those things and trying to understand where they're coming from. I think collectively, the Autistic community need to be very much empowered. We need to find our strength and power and know who we are. I feel strongly it's not enough just to include people, inclusion just to look good. That's not good enough. It's being genuine and authentic of our strengths. We're brought forth by our strength. It doesn't matter whoever we are, we all have our strengths. No matter where we belong, we're bringing something, bringing our healing, healing for family. It's important for our ways of to be respected.

I still come up against some blocks when I try to work outside my profession, my nursing profession. Yes, I have my Nursing degree and licence. It's not an issue. But when I go outside my creative field, the work is challenging, very challenging. They notice very quickly that you are on the spectrum and very quickly you are picked on by people who don't understand you're different and everything changes. That's still happening. At the moment that's singing. I'm trying to move into that area as a newbie. It's really moving into personal challenges. It's coming up against all the belief system and blocks people have about you as part of these things.

There needs to be a real change. That's how I feel and I do still feel deeply about the world, the planet, especially people's consciousness. I want to see a shift from the assumptions. We all move forward as one. Definitely, that's the goal.'

I will also talk about finding my voice. I'm very grateful and I'm very lucky to have found my voice. This is the voice that has taken years to find. I was always able to speak. So I suppose it's not to get me wrong. I think I was always supposed to fight my way through things, or maybe fight for what I wanted or what I needed. I wasn't empowered. I was largely disempowered, like being in the bottom of a well and shouting and fighting my way up for what I need or feel in the darkness, like no real strength behind it because I didn't really know who I was or what I was even fighting for. As such, there's the inner self, and the subconscious I guess. I hadn't realised that there was an empowerment needed in life. I didn't know that I was disempowered.

Not everyone will have a voice, not everyone finds it easy to express themselves, or to explain to people what it is like on the Autism Spectrum, how it is for them. Some people are good at it, some people are very articulate. Some people could learn and we have some non-verbal people who are really good at writing and expressing it that way.

It can be a huge challenge for people on the spectrum to try and explain what's going on. So I suppose, I'm taking up the challenge in myself really and for myself. It's still a challenge to express to you all how it is, being in my body to do what I'm doing, how it has been in my own life. I suppose I'm using myself because it's the only 100% definition I'm sure of in my life of how I was. I can't speak for others. When I was a young child, I didn't speak that much. I feel like I was consciously humanitarian always. We all have that instinct in us. Some people are stronger than others in what is right, what's fair and what's good and what's not. And that was very much in my awareness. So I would have always wondered why there was so much injustice and injustice and injustice. I suddenly know it's everywhere.

But at the same time, there's such beauty. As I grew and grew in self awareness, becoming knowing and understanding, then you see the beauty in everything. Now, I choose the beauty. I don't choose to see the darkness. You hold the awareness of what you can transform and that there's duality in everything, everything. There's nothing that doesn't have a duality including myself, everyone. There's a duality in everything and everyone and we are all part of this. I suppose terms of life.

So as the awareness and knowing of that came through, then I see more. And instead of complaining of the injustices and expanding on the injustices that are there, it's just to face them head-on. Maybe transmutation, transform the thinking about them and then we will see them dissolve. That's the only way I can explain that. By looking at it and accepting it, it can be transformed.

Look at myself, when I had the diagnosis, I'm looking at it, going through all that, healing, then accepting eventually that this is what it is. So communication to me is a huge thing. It's not that I want to sit behind videos everyday. But it's because I had no where else to say what I needed to say in the past. And in the last few years, the desire to go behind the screen and speak it out and say it out was there.

The desire is there because you realise that you can and that you can explain to people how it is in reality. That is important. It is important for so many people around the world diagnosed with Autism. There are a lot of them who will not have the awareness to speak and let people know what they want. Other people need to be doing this, making transformations that are very needed. There's a need for a new understanding of the intelligence that we all share of how that is and not just what is assumed.

So it's good that we are open to learn from each other. That's the most important thing for me, having my page, writing my book. It's about learning for myself and others. As I speak, I'm learning more. It's all transformation and growth.

CHAPTER TWO

ASPERGER SYNDROME – INVISIBLE CHALLENGES AND HIDDEN GIFTS

It is a neurodevelopmental condition affecting communication and social interaction, and those with the condition having repetitive and/or stereotypical behaviours and limited interests. However as well as this many people can excel in particular areas to varying degrees, some displaying savant and genius attributes.

My own story is definitely one of coming out of darkness in many ways and into light. Asperger's has been an invisible challenge for much of my life, but also a transformative one, because many hidden gifts have surfaced through a process of developing self-awareness. To give a brief history I was born in the countryside in a very peaceful and quiet area. Being the youngest in the family and the only girl I spent much time with the animals we had, along with doing simple things such as playing with dolls as a young child. I enjoyed my own company in many ways, and in a world I had essentially created for myself.

I attended mainstream primary and secondary schools and then at 23 I completed a Bachelor of Science in mental health nursing at the University of Limerick from 2002 to 2006.

I have experienced anxiety, depression and panic attacks, all to varying degrees. But in the last 3 years they have remarkably reduced. Depressive episodes are 1 to 2 a year now and not as severe. Panic attacks have disappeared, and I don't feel anxiety except on a rare occasion. Overall I feel the work I have done on myself and continue to do daily has paid off. I believe this can also be the case for others. Doing personal self-awareness work in this way could also lead to not having a dependence on medication in the long term. This is my personal opinion. There are of course people who will need to remain stable on medication. Here it is invaluable.

I've adopted the attitude that I shall take what I need from every course, person, experience, book etc. but I will ultimately do what's best for me and use what works for me.

I'd like to share the ways in which I was helped to overcome much of the confusion, depression and anxiety of the past to where I am now, which is a place of quiet knowing of myself in so many ways that I continue to discover every day what makes me grateful for this gift of life that I have been given and the gift of people in my life that make it all worthwhile. I am truly lucky and blessed.

I could write chapters on the events that changed my life but for now I will put into bullet points what worked and what continues to work for me to improve my overall health, mood, and day to day life. If this helps even 1 person then it is always worthwhile.

Mentorship – I can't stress enough the value of mentors in any way shape or form to guide people forward and as well as helping to motivate and assist people push past limitations. I personally have had at least 5 to 6 mentors in my life in different areas that have motivated me in numerous ways.

Self-awareness – There are so many books out there around this subject of cultivating self-awareness but ultimate self-awareness comes from within. Do some research on how you can develop this for yourself. It could be through journaling, reflection, a mindfulness practice, counselling, Cognitive Behavioural Therapy etc. The list goes on. All of value. Find what works for you and keep doing it.

Meditation – When I began to attempt to meditate my concentration span was zero. It was difficult. Now I am available to teach meditation groups and do so from time to time. Obviously this is ten years down the line from when I attempted it first. Keep trying and don't give up on it. The benefits are life changing.

Physical Exercise – Depending of course on a person's health and deemed fit by a doctor. I go to the gym as regularly as possible. I too have days that it's hard to motivate myself, but I always feel better afterwards and that knowledge gets me up and out. Anything that gets the body moving is good – dance, walking, sport.

Vitamins – Again best to make sure there are no contraindications to any medications you are taking, but what I find especially good are B vitamins, plus a multivitamin, minerals, udos oil, seeds, fruit and vegetables and adequate protein in the diet.

Gratitude – The more grateful we are for what we have the more we will have to be grateful for. No matter how bad things feel or seem. There's always something to be grateful for. That said at times it can be difficult when people suffer depression. But don't forget that this too shall pass and while you're in that space be good to yourself and seek out a support of some sort. Eg www.grow.ie or www.aware.ie who offer great support.

Love – There is always someone on this planet who loves you and who you love. For me I am lucky to have the love of family, my children who are 17 and 16 now and have lived this journey along with me their whole lives, and the support of a great man who came into my life almost a year ago. I accept that every day will be different and every day we will grow and learn, no matter what comes our way.

In conclusion, I feel that although there have been challenges in that Asperger Syndrome can be invisible outwardly to others (which can be difficult when people have expectations of you fitting in to normal everyday situations) but I would say to anyone with Asperger Syndrome to be yourself and nurture your own gifts and talents that can be hidden at times.

I am lucky enough to have had people believe in my abilities along the way, for example in my innate healing abilities which I have been encouraged to develop, all helping me to realise the depth of the gifts I've been given. I'm also singing now and am being mentored and helped in recent times to get out there and never give up. Much time and effort is being put into this by my husband who is an accomplished musician and teacher, so thank you!

I would love to create a CD to raise money for Autism Charities in Limerick and Ireland and hopefully that will come about. If there are people who are interested in helping with this, whether they'd like to contribute to the CD or help to create it, that would be great. Feel free to email me via paulanash0@gmail.com

I am hugely grateful for every mentor who has helped me, and also to everyone who has said 'no' to me, as they all helped me to find my way.

CHAPTER THREE

STIMMING

From an autistic point of view, I want to get across what I feel this is. These are my feelings as a person who is on the spectrum. Stimming is self soothing. It's regulation, emotional regulation. It's mental regulation, it's spiritual as well as physical. It can work in different ways but all of that is a need to regulate and also because we are so over stimulated from the environment. Generally, to help with understanding, we on the autism spectrum are probably a 100 times more overstimulated than a neurotypical person depending on the environment and etc.

So it's important to be able to regulate the environments that are out of our control and also environments that are over stimulating or under stimulating. It really depends. I think it comes in different ways. I want to bring it to more normalization. Brushing my hair is a stim. Not brushing it just once but to continue brushing it. I like flicking it, twirling it or touching it because my hair is long. When I got older, I discovered exciting things like make-up, and hair extensions, braids. I started to get them, putting them into my hair because I like the weight of it in my hair, the hair straightener is a huge tool. I could just be straightening my hair and keep going over and over. That's a stim too. You may find some people continue to change their hair in different styles. All of this is stimming in different ways. Obviously, it's more extreme with us.

I'm sure normal everyday people also stim in different ways a little bit maybe. For us, it's a way of life. It's who we are. It's part of our being innately and this is done often unconsciously.

There are things when I do them, I realise that it's stimming; repetitive action movements like finger flicking, nail tapping on a table. You could see people chew pens. It could be two different extremes. I wasn't a pen chewer but yes you could tap a pencil, tap objects on a surface. This is done mostly to hear a repetitive noise. All of these I will class as everyday stims as people may not have any other thing to use.

Also dance movements, it could be dance, or shaking movement or meditation that would be repetitive enough. It will open up and bring me to the place where I would end up clapping or singing, I have echolalia. I also love chants.

Ultimately, it's around regulation, around joy and excitement. You can feel it come into your body. You can be excited and be yourself. You let go and not mask. Stimming could be a way to express joy, excitement. It can be about stress too. Sometimes if you are stressed and it's all built up and you can't get it out or you are in a situation where you have to mask everything inside you, you might stim to ease all the pressure. Some people might head bang even though it can be injurious. For the person, they don't feel the pain at the moment. This injurious behaviour would need to be monitored. There is a risk of injury. People should be helped and managed in certain situations without harming the person. But it's still to be done without interfering with the person, without harming the person, without burdening, without judgment.

This is important when it comes to stimming in different situations and different extremes. Some people could stim all day. That is the way for them, for some of us who feel the urge to do it. Again it depends on situations. Is it at work or at home?

Looking back on my childhood and things that I used to enjoy as stims would be spinning, spinning your body around circles in different directions. It's very soothing, very relaxing. That was fun and it was also a stim. Also going on the children's swings in the forest a few miles from where we lived was stimming. In other ways, rocking is also a stim. I wouldn't do it unless I'm completely under stress. Finger flicking, hand movements, body movements, all repetitive body movements can be stims. All of these bring back regulation, they help to emotionally regulate, and help to be calm.

It's important for people on the spectrum, people who are autistic to be able to stim without being interfered with by other people, without people trying to stop them, trying to control them. I feel that when people are prevented and stopped and bullied, it makes it much harder for them to be in control internally. There's really no need for people to bully autistic children and adults in any setting whatsoever. This is beyond comprehension and it is wrong. I feel strongly about it. Everyone is individual. Every autistic person is a unique individual. It is important to respect them even if you don't understand them, even if they are different, and not considered neurotypical.

There's an inner reason why stimming is done. I feel it's in our bodies. You may not understand the level of overwhelming stress, overwhelming sensory overload people can have. The same with the other end of the spectrum where people don't feel it the way we do. You can't just go on Google and type one line on stimming and say everybody is under the heading now who's on the autistic spectrum. These are my thoughts and feelings about stimming. Another autistic person may have a different view on stimming but that is perfectly okay. I'm just speaking for myself. I'm not speaking for the entire community. But I'm sure we share a lot of similarities.

CHAPTER FOUR

MASKING, BOUNDARIES

MASKING

One of the real positive things about coming out as an autistic person in my opinion is not really having to mask your personality. When you no longer mask, you are not as tired or exhausted or burnt out as you would have been in the past. In the past, if I was going to work, if you are going anywhere, if you are going to meet people, the mask you put on could turn you into some sort of a chameleon and you just join in with whatever you are at and whoever you are with. You learn to just mesh with others and be like them so as to fit and get along with people.

It's a huge relief not to have to do that anymore if I'm honest, although it has come to a stage where you don't have friends lining out at the door waiting to go out with you or waiting to connect with you because now, everything has changed. You have become real, you have become who you are, you are not going to fit in or try to fit in with people because you just know that you are beyond that.

I can't go back and be the person I was before, the chameleon, the doormat type of person I was in so many ways. I think when you grow past that and you realise who you are, what you like, what you don't like, what your needs are, what helps you to stay, what helps you in this world, you feel much better as a person.

There's so much thrown out there these days, a huge sensory overload for somebody who is sensitive. There are people who are so sensitive and it's not worth it using up every piece of your energy just to please other people, just to appear like a normal everyday person. I don't feel it's right.

I'm in a happy space in my life with that. But there has been sacrifices along the way as well and it hasn't come easy. You are always at the risk of being misunderstood when actually you are just protecting yourself, your energy, creating your own boundaries. That's an entitlement that we have as a people, everyone has.

Sometimes, I feel we just need to get to know ourselves. The good news is that I don't need to mask anymore, even if I really try to mask, it doesn't happen. But it can be tough for other people because I'm myself with no kind of apology. I won't make any apology for who I am or my way of being. If that's tough for some people, then there's a reason for that. That's something they might look at for themselves.

There are so many people on the spectrum who don't realise that they are masking, like it was for me. Hopefully what we do and what we share and what I'm putting out here will help someone someway or the other. I don't have a huge agenda. This is more about being able to speak because it's a good thing to do, it's a powerful place to be in and it's nice to share about. Hopefully other people will step into their own truth and empowerment.

BOUNDARIES

I would also talk about boundaries from the point of view of someone who has had to put boundaries in place over quite a long period of time and who at one point didn't even know what boundaries were. I would give a brief on what they are for me now. I feel boundaries. I know they are important.

Mental, Emotional and Physical boundaries. Most of us have different beliefs. Whatever it is, you are entitled to that belief system and that feeling as well as the boundary around it. You are entitled to that whether people agree with you or not, whether they make sense or not, whether it's right or wrong. There's a boundary around that. My belief is my own and people don't have to agree with it. They can think I'm completely off the wall. It doesn't affect me or bother me. That's the boundary that I have. I'm entitled to my spiritual beliefs, the path that I'm on, what I feel has helped me change my life and to transcend a lot of things that were holding me back. That's my own belief system and that's what worked for me. I believe in God, in everything like omnipresent, transcendence. I'm not going to push my beliefs on others. I am connected to God, to the Holy Spirit energy, and to Christ Light energy. I also enjoy the energy of the forest and being by the ocean. There's power and beauty in everything depending on how you look at it. That's the boundary that I have and if people don't like my beliefs and the way I feel, that's okay. It doesn't mean that we can't get on. It doesn't mean that I wouldn't hold firm in my own feelings.

I just see it that everyone is entitled to their opinions, their beliefs, to whatever system they were brought up in, or to whatever that transcends and moves through for them. It's individual. We are on a journey. Everyone is where they are on that journey and judgment isn't helpful because we were all in a different place before and we have all moved through stuff. We are constantly evolving, we are constantly growing. I just think it's important to hold on to our boundaries and what's right for us.

Moving on to mental boundaries, I feel a mental boundary is a boundary around our individual way of thinking, right or wrong. My ideas and feelings and what I think about are my own. I feel they don't need to be inspected especially by those close in my life. They don't have to agree. That's fine. My thoughts are my own, how I feel about things and how I think as a person are my unique attributes. It doesn't make it right or wrong. It's the same with everyone else. And I respect that everyone else has a way of thinking that might not be shared with me. I feel it's very important to have boundaries where people can't tell you how to think. It's really important that we are allowed the space to think for ourselves, be free thinkers, free beings in the world and to exercise the right to be free thinking people. Obviously, I don't advocate for us to harm ourselves or others in the process. I just feel we do our best everyday with the way we think, and how we use what we think about because thoughts are also powerful entities themselves. The more you think about some things, the more they are going to come into form sooner or later, one way or the other. Some thoughts may be faster than others. That's the way it is. That's how I feel. Maybe it's a belief but I have known it to be true.

So mental boundaries are around the way of thinking and treating yourself and not harming others in the process. I'm free in that.

Emotional boundaries is around our emotions, how we feel about situations, people and so on. Our feelings are important in the sense that I'm entitled to my feelings even if other people don't agree or other people think I'm crazy or mad. I'm entitled to my feelings, my emotions and I also have a responsibility for how I act on them and what I create around them. Knowing the power of emotions and how they can affect other people and learning in those ways is important. I think having boundaries around what I feel about things is safe. It's responsible. It's protective. It's important that they are respected. My emotional state and wellbeing are very important. I have been through a lot emotionally in life. I have learned to regulate my emotions at this point much better than what I would have done years ago, 10 years ago even. I feel that's a shift in my own life and the awareness of my emotional state is very important to me, the same as the awareness of other states of being. It helps me to navigate life. Boundaries are vital.

Physical boundaries, a lot of people can say that's simple. But in some ways, it's not because a lot of communication is done nonverbally and things are unsaid a lot of the time. If you move into a room with a crowd of people using the period of covid for example and somebody just walks away from somebody because they are uncomfortable or someone is at fault, it's obviously a bodily physical boundary being exhibited. We feel the right to feel safe and to feel secure in situations. I feel a lot of physical boundaries are non-verbal and it can be helpful to have more awarenesses of what physical boundaries are. Physical boundaries can change depending on situations, the people involved, the relationships involved. All of that is interchangeable. It's not just black and white. Any boundary you have with somebody can be loosened and changed depending the evolution of trust within the relationship and the evolution of the relationship itself.

I wouldn't say everything is black and white. There's always a grey area where you can stay where you are with somebody. You look at a friendship you have with somebody and how you see the evolution and the boundaries spiritually, mentally, emotionally and physically. It's good to look at it. Some people look at their intimate relationship with partners but they don't necessarily look at their friendships with friends at different levels. That's important, also acquaintances, co-workers, bosses and so on. Every connection affects us in some way.

Group settings like work situations also require boundaries for you to be who you are and be happy within yourself at that work. I'm trying to navigate through the broadness of boundaries. We learn to speak out more rather than having everything unsaid. In the process, we become more open, more vocal when something isn't right. It's important especially for young people like people under 18 and even elderly people. There's a lot of vulnerability. There are different types of scenarios which would require different types of boundaries.

I feel it's a broad area and I have learned so much about it in the past few years. It has really uplifted my own life. It has uplifted my sense of well being and sense of autonomy over my own life and space that I'm in and the space that I decide to share with other people.

It's very much about choosing. I just don't have everything happen to me. I create thoughts, actions, words in my life and I'm very conscious of my desires and everything playing out in my life. I'm living it. You keep to it as much as you can, we have no control over other people. We can only control ourselves but I feel that the more we bring the positives into things, the more we accept the sense of not having control over the actions of others and accept more responsibility for our own actions. Then we draw more positivity to ourselves and also the right people who respect us and our boundaries will remain and stay in our lives. Those that choose otherwise will be more at a distance and those who choose to keep pushing our boundaries will also be kept more at a distance. That just seems like the way it plays out. It's important, it's freedom and eliminates confusion. It eliminates not being able to name friendships, relationships, not being able to decide how you feel about things. It becomes much clearer. We are able to decide what we want, what we are willing to accept and what we are not willing to accept, this is what we are leaving behind and this is what we are moving forward with.

When things don't feel right in my heart, my energy, or my soul, I'm free to walk away. I think when you get stronger, you just want to live a positive and happy life as much as you can.

There's a duality to everything. We can create things and they become real. Life becomes very real and the truth becomes magnified and amplified, and gratefully accepted.

Everyone has got to figure out their own way with boundaries in their own lives with people that are around them but starting off with themselves, then with connections. Then moving out to examine other connections. You will start to realise where you are at with all of this. Is your life being lived through you? Are you creating your life yourself? Or is it just happening. Are you the one moving the energy and creating situations and so on? Nothing is meant to be without us having a part in it, in the creation of it. It makes sense to me. I have been living it and having been mentored in a lot of ways myself by amazing people who brought out that truth in me. Hopefully by speaking about it, it will bring out the truth for others as well. All my hopes and wishes are to share what I have gained and learned. If it suits certain people, then great.

CHAPTER FIVE

EATING DISORDERS

Let's look at eating disorders, disordered eating in association with Autism. I will use myself as an example because it's the easiest way to try to explain the feeling around food and textures and sensory issues.

Now, I have gained self awareness more so around what I do. You start having certainty of what you are doing and why you are doing it, why you are eating and why you are not eating. From my own experience, I have a love of certain foods. I don't like every type of food. I like the experience of eating, the pleasure of eating. It's like another addiction or drugs. Food is no different in my opinion.

In my experience with alcohol, with cigarettes, with whatever gives people pleasure, I always love food. I just don't like to eat animals but that was more of a choice than an aversion. It wasn't that I had dislike of the taste of it. I lived on a farm, the animals were like people to me. I was always like that even as a small child. I feel maybe not necessarily because I have Autism. It was always a choice.

From when I was small l, I've always loved vegetables, potatoes. If I had a choice and being honest about it, I would mash up all of my food and I love juice as well. I like them liquid. I like the sensory experience. I try to explain it so that people might get an idea of how it could be for somebody. Liquid pureed food, mashed-up, gravies, sauces, things that make it easier to swallow and to ingest the food.

I wouldn't be keen on eating fruits just like eating them out of my hand. I prefer them juiced. That's just something personal to me. There are a lot of people on the spectrum who are the exact opposite of me. They wouldn't be able to eat anything that I eat.

The awareness should be held when you are looking at people, looking at small kids being looked after and they are on the spectrum and people are trying to force feed them. Maybe, they have an aversion or their body can't take this particular food at that particular time. They just don't like it and I think it's important you could try it a few times but if it keeps happening, it's important to respect that the child might not like that type of food. I'm somebody who would not be happy to see people being forced fed or being made to eat certain food. I think it's important to look at the children as individuals and get to know them even by body language because most of the communication most of the time whether we talk or not is non verbal especially if you can't fully communicate or if you have issues around communication.

So if you are working with special needs children who are on the spectrum, it's important to look and ask, "Do they want to eat the food? Is this good for them?" That's one issue. Sensory issues with food is huge. Now, I have the awareness of the insight when I go shopping to look at what I'm doing, what I'm buying and why I'm buying it. I'm not just buying whatever everyone else wants to buy to eat it because everyone else is eating it.

Now, I have decided that I'm going to eat the way I want to eat at this stage, what fits my body and what is right for me.

Also, food intolerance is a thing. People on the spectrum might not be able to tolerate certain foods. When I had a food intolerance done a few years ago, I was quite surprised at what showed up because I was eating and drinking many things I was intolerant to. I was intolerant to tomatoes, to bananas, to coffee, cocoa. I was intolerant to alcohol after drinking for years and not knowing. I think there's a huge importance around finding out.

Say you have a child on the spectrum that is having trouble eating, maybe find out if they are intolerant to certain foods and it will help everyone. At the end of the day, it will help the child not to feel stressed and it will help the parents not to feel stressed. It opens up more reality around what we can eat and what we can't eat. Often, the taste can be much stronger for us. You can have situations where you are just not able to eat certain foods. You wouldn't want to be forced. If someone ever tried to force me to eat something, it would be the first and last time.

As an adult on the spectrum, you can control the cravings. I get a lot of food cravings.

I think it's something people can look at and take in when they are working with people, adults, children or you are the one involved. You have to look at your own preference, look at why you are eating something, what you are drawn to, what you are craving and maybe what emotional associations it may have. It can be subconscious rather than conscious.

So I'll say, look at your emotions, look at why you are doing what you are doing. It's a great way of having insight into first of all on yourself and second of all other people. So when you are doing your food shop, have a look at what you are buying, why you are buying it and look at what you used to like as a child, maybe you stopped eating something. Were you force fed? A lot people think it's a good idea to keep trying. It's not an intentional forced feeding scenario. A lot of parents just try keep trying to get the child eat vegetables and think it might be more healthy. But I think if a child eats anything, it's good.

Then you can have people having fixations around food. People can go through a lot of things in their minds that they might not speak about at all. People might be fixated or have thoughts around foods. Maybe it's a way of control, like it's often a control mechanism. If people feel out of control in their lives, they are going to sit back and try and find something to control. So often it can be food because people can control what they put in their body and etcetera. They might not have control of the broader experience of their lives, especially teenagers, they go through a lot. An autistic teenager goes through a huge amount of stress because they have hormones and peer pressure and trying to find out who they are.

This is one of the things to look at to open up conversation around it with them because they might not even realise it themselves. It could be a sub-conscious trait.

Textures, some people might like soft foods, other people might like raw, hard foods. It's just individual. I was lucky enough as a person and as a professional to work in the area of eating disorders, I worked in this area twice for 6 months each time. It's a residential centre. It was really variable in the clients that were there.

Again, like a lot of clients that come into these residential eating disorder centres, they might not be openly on the spectrum. There might be a few, there might be those who are not aware. I'm not saying everyone is. Of course not. But there are probably people who are not aware and they are joining the eating disorder programmes. They are trying to battle these disorders. They don't really know why they have a disorder with foods. Some people are anorexic and some bulimic and there are people suffering binge eating disorder and other unspecified eating disorders. It was really fascinating to me and I walked on some of the journey with them, and heard their different stories and different ways of being.

I have disordered eating patterns. It depends on the levels of stress in my life. I won't say I'm fully a binge disordered person. Though there were times I would have been but I don't think it's always the same. It can be restricting as well at times. It depends. I have never made myself sick though, I couldn't do that. That's something I wouldn't be able to do. There are a lot of people who are not like me. There are a lot of people who don't want to eat. It can be because of self loathing, people who just do not want to live. You have so many different scenarios. I've seen so many scenarios that I can't say this person is on the spectrum or that person. All i can say though is that the model used where I was was very good. But I felt that if you are an autistic person and someone is bringing you food blindly and you don't know what you will be getting for lunch or dinner, it's very tough. It's part of this program and you are expected to eat it. It's a very stressful situation to be in. When you have no choice in what is going to be cooked for you, this can be challenging. I think the program is very good. But there's room for improvement in programs for people with Autism and to lessen the stress of what is expected especially if you are paying for the program to get well.

I would urge professionals to look again at the Autistic person and the difference. So as to develop individual programs and keep it open to develop programs that might work across the board, there's a need for more understanding.

I will say that if I was somebody who couldn't verbalize what I wanted, and I was pushed into an institution, I wouldn't like it. I've worked in many different institutions, 16 years nursing and I was a care assistant for 6 years prior. I have worked with many Autistic people at a time I didn't know I was, I've come in contact with many people in the course of my work, verbal and nonverbal people, watching what's going on as a professional and now obviously at a deeper level of knowing. I've always been empathetic. I always felt for people in different scenarios but I would feel there needs to be a change in how things are done, how people are fed, how people are expected to eat and how the pharmaceutical side is being handled as well.

Looking at people in residential centres, there might be a child who might be nonverbal; the routine is getting up in the morning, bringing them out, they get fed, they are brought back to wherever like the sitting room. I think what is given often doesn't digest. Some people don't tolerate it and there is a laxative prescribed for these people as well on top of that. I will not go into the negative side. I like to focus on the positives. But at the same time, the truth will always be the truth.

There's really a need for change in how people are trained, in how staff are trained to look after people in these situations. It's a lack of education more than anything because people are only doing what they are seeing. People are trained to do something, they are going to do it because they don't know any difference unless they are experienced themselves or their family member or friend already had the experience.

It's not a blame game but it's important to have a change from the top down on how things are done. To do that, there needs to be understanding of what needs to change, how it feels to be on the other side of the fence.

I still go around as I'm an agency nurse and I go into different situations as often as possible. I like to move around in different places, see different things. It's not that I'm there to spy on people. I'm there to do my best as a professional. But as things happen and I see things, then I would say something. I would attempt to change it.

I see it's hard to get in and change things and even because I'm out as an autistic person. Everywhere I go to work, I'm not masking, they do know very quickly who or what I am or they have an idea maybe. Often it hasn't been taken very well coming from me if I say something. But I'm not going to stop telling the truth about us.

At the end of the day, I don't see it as intentional. I see it as people not really knowing any better. We do what we can. These people inspire us to come out and say things better.

As I said, if I could have my diet pureed and liquidized, I'll go along and do it. I guess that's why I used to like alcohol and that was part of the problem, the addiction that I had.

If you have children on the spectrum or you are on the spectrum yourself, it's good to sit and examine foods, your relationship with foods. Why do I want to eat or not eat? Do I want to eat because I'm feeling this emotional hole? Is there something going on subconsciously, emotionally that I'm not even aware of? As Autistics, we can go through a lot of emotions and not be aware of them. It can take me 24 hours to process something that someone says to me now. I know how I feel about things, that's a personal thing. Other people can be different.

You can ask yourself why am I eating? Why am I starving myself? Why am I controlling my food situation? A lot of these can control us. We can't often control things. So until we can come into more empowerment, change might be difficult. A lot of people don't have the luxury of empowerment because there are a lot of things against them. It can be very hard for them to rise as especially when people don't expect them to rise.

I have not worked with younger children. I have only worked with 16 years old and older. I know there are many young kids in different hospitals with eating disorders and on different programs. I'm sure there are many who are autistic and many who have different spectrum traits and co-morbidities Within myself, my work teaches me a lot about my own journey and the way I am with food.

CHAPTER SIX

GENUINE INCLUSION

I want to articulate my vision about what I can see for the present. Awareness and acceptance etc. Firstly, awareness is important. It's important to bring a sense of respect into that. Being aware of something that that person over there is autistic. I'm aware. I'm aware that this group of people here are autistic. But just because I'm aware doesn't mean that I understand, it doesn't mean that I know what to do next. It doesn't mean that I'm going to know how to interact with these people. So I understand that being an autistic person, other people can find it tough and they really don't know how to react to us or even know how to speak to us, how to initiate conversation because I feel there's a lack of education around this in a sense now education is coming out, we are coming out. I am speaking about what we need.

A lot of people are writing about autism, they are writing about autistic people but they haven't experienced what it is like to live our lives, to be us, to really know what we need, rather than assuming. Basically, there are assumptions made about autistic people and people don't know any other way to relate except what they have learned or read.

From my point of view, awareness is a great thing. It's great to be aware that somebody in the room is autistic. But what to do next? There has to be more than this awareness. Self awareness is the key. We can have awareness for our selves but talk different things. Self awareness is a big difference. It's fabulous.

How do we interconnect this awareness and this knowing? Somebody working with us is autistic, so what next? It's education. We can educate the society and educate the world. We are trying to do this, a lot of us know how it is, what we need and what we don't need. We are just everyday normal people. We may live in a different way. We are still normal. I consider myself a normal person. I'm here in the world. I live in my own way and I have my own way of doing things. But I'm no different in my feelings and emotions than anyone else, in the desires I have, in what I want in my life or what I want for myself.

There's a gap that needs to be bridged around that. So awareness is a great thing.

We are part of society, part of community, we are in schools, we are in workplaces. We might have to work a bit harder than some other people. But we are there. That's important to try and articulate that is a challenge for me at the moment. That's my feeling.

Instead of just awareness, we are respected for who we are, what we represent as a people. We are respected as individuals as well because we are not all the same. We are different like any other human being. It needs to be genuine respect. Genuine respect is a huge thing. So if somebody is pretending to respect you because it looks good to others, because they think this is something I need to try and do for whatever reason, then that is totally ingenuine, and that is not going to work because we do know when someone is genuine with you or not or how someone changes with you.

Before I was diagnosed, I worked with people and I know what it's like to be treated with respect because they didn't know I was autistic. And that's not to say that everybody changed after that. But a lot of people changed, I have to be honest. A lot of people changed after they found out and you are treated differently. I really was surprised.

It was an interesting awakening because I got to realise the extent of people's beliefs around it, lack of simple education around it and I sat back and said, 'wow'. I couldn't believe there's so many different levels of reaction to me as an autistic person. In the future and in the present, I feel that when we come out, we should not have to deal with other people's projections as well as our own healing and belief systems that don't belong to us at all. Awareness is fantastic but there should be more depth to it.

Acceptance is a beautiful thing. But there's a lot of mixed reaction around acceptance. From the point of view of my own journey, acceptance of myself, coming from an unknowing and coming from a space where I thought I was somebody else, someone I had created to fit in, I didn't really know who I was. Then coming into acceptance of myself was a challenge because I didn't know who I was to begin with and I felt would I have made certain choices in my life if I had known? Would I have become a nurse? But the answer is yes. I would have because I had years to come into the knowing of myself and really figure out who I am.

I realised that everything that I chose career wise was there for me. That was never going to be any different. But it took me a long time to achieve self acceptance because I came out like that into the society. I wouldn't say there wasn't acceptance but people are aware of you and I found it fascinating in some ways and unsettling at the same time in other ways because I was vulnerable. As to the reaction, I felt like an alien that has just landed here and people talk to you like you are five years old. These things I feel need to change, there needs to be a shift around that. People don't really have to go through that and they don't have to be the elephant in the room just because they are autistic.

It's really the wider society and our own community coming into full acceptance of ourselves, who we are , what we stand for together and individually and with the general society. There needs to be acceptance all over. It's not just about putting it out there and saying we want to be accepted.

With awareness there has to be a follow up on that. It's agendaless so that people are not pretending to accept you. It's a journey and in time, there's no need to put it out there even till we come to a point where we are beyond that, where we all accept ourselves, our journey, each other and the society and individuals. That will happen. There are a lot of vulnerable members of our society that some of us are speaking out on their behalf in a way. But they have their own feelings and ideas as well. Some people just can't articulate it. Some may develop and articulate later in future time.

Advocating is a tight rope because I am not everyone. I don't stand for everyone on the spectrum. I'm an autistic person in my own right but I'm not speaking for everyone. It's around protecting the vulnerable people but also promoting the path of empowerment, for myself, for other people, for the wider society. There needs to be genuiness in the wider society around genuinely wanting to connect with us, not just because they are told they should accept.

I feel that at this stage in my life I'm in acceptance of who I am. I don't need anyone else to accept me in order to do what I do, live as I live and so on. But not everyone feels like that. I have come to that point because I worked for everything. I have emotionally, spiritually, not just in the way of physical work. I have worked on myself as well. I won't allow that to be undervalued. That is how I feel about acceptance.

Acceptance is not just being accepted but valued for who we are in diverse terms, valued for what we can bring to the workplaces, to the society, to anything we are engaged. That we are actually seen as valuable and that our opinion, the way we work, whatever it is, whatever we can offer is valuable and is not going to be dismissed.

People have to be willing to hear what we have to say. That's a huge thing. That's important.

Ultimately, inclusion. Inclusion in everything in life , in school, in workplaces, in society is important to us. Genuine inclusion. There are autistic people who need reasonable accommodations. That has to be allowed in the workplace. A reasonable accommodation is not just like a wheelchair. It goes much further than that with the sensory issues people have. People on the spectrum have a lot of different needs and they vary hugely depending on the individual. Some people have meltdowns if they are very overloaded and all of these need to be understood.

I think people need to come in and help us with the way of doing these things and creating space for it. The same with schools that are for nonverbal people etc. including nonverbal adults and different institutions. There's a lot of work that is needed to be done to help staff understand as well that these people are valuable and just because these people don't speak doesn't mean that they do not feel things the way we do.

There's still an unconsciousness Sometimes, we all need to be reminded that there's more to these people than what is set on the worklist, or what is written about them. There's more to it than that. I feel strongly about it because there's more to be learned for all of us. There is more to be learned for all of us. Inclusion in every way is important.

Empowerment is a huge thing. This has to come from within. It's something we must do for ourselves if we can. In whatever way people can be empowered, there can be so many different ways. That has to come from within ultimately and also with help from others if necessary. But with the view that somebody is capable themselves and they know what they want and they know how they want it. They don't have to be told what to do. You have to believe that Autistic people know what they want to do, know what they don't want, know our limits and know how to regulate ourselves in different ways.

If people need more help, we have to know that there is a boundary and autistic people have a right to their space as well as to their dignity.

I believe in the goodness of people, a lot of people came in to help me normal everyday people, different types of people. I have seen a lot of goodness in people. I believe that it is possible. I believe that because ultimately we are one.

I believe it's going to be possible for us all to rise up and come together, moving forward from both communities. There's a shift that is happening. There will be a wider shift in the next few years. From there, things will be much easier for the people coming out after us hopefully.

A lot still needs to change because a lot of autistic people are still suffering. People want to try and cure them, change them. I don't need to be cured or changed. I'm quite happy and content the way I am.

I really find it distressing that people can actually believe that at this point in time in the 21st century. I find it hard to sit back and not come out and speak because of things like that. Now, I don't focus on the negatives. I would rather focus on the positives. That doesn't mean that I'm not aware of everything that is going on. It just means that I'm not willing to focus on them.

Empowerment is about focusing on and enhancing our strengths, what we can see that can be improved, what we can see in people that is good, how to positively come out and educate people on as much as we can about our diversity, the way we think, the way we see things and divisions we have. That's very important.

We do have a lot of visions that when taken seriously, when we are actually valued, respected and brought into the society without us asking for this are highly valuable. That is the dawning that is coming. It's here in the 'now' and I believe it will prevail and we will sit equally and be able to help each other out. From education to running the country, we are capable. We all have things we can bring to the table that maybe people are not aware of or haven't thought of. As an autistic person, if I put my mind on something, it's 100% on that and that's where we achieve our goals and aims. We can work completely for that specific goal and we can put all our energy into this whereas some people may struggle with that.

From my point of view, autism is not solely about charity or deficit. It completely depends on the individual and situation at hand. We are there with the same value as anyone else. We might just work differently. Acceptance is the first step, then moving into unity with other people, it all starts from within, so what we feel in ourselves, we see it more outside and we need to be strong as a community as well. Those of us who are autistic need to become strong enough to stand solid in who we are and know we do deserve respect and we deserve to feel valued. After acceptance, we are moving into respect, inclusion, empowerment and so on and so forth. It's all about the whole picture and it must be genuine.

CHAPTER SEVEN

ANXIETY AND DEPRESSION

I would like to talk about anxiety and I would like to use myself as an example. Anxiety is rooted in fear. When you look at it from a broader perspective, you look at what it actually is. Anxiety is fear, fear of anything. But the fear a lot of the time means we are not present. If you are in fear and you are suffering from anxiety then obviously, you are not in the 'Now'.

Maybe your worrying is about a past event that happened, or you are worrying about something that is coming in the future. Whatever that may be, the root of it is fear. A young child will present differently, they will be uncomfortable or unsettled, cry or have different behaviours. The fear can present depending on how comfortable you are in a situation. If a child or a baby is uncomfortable in a situation, they might not be aware that they have anxiety. They might be aware they are fearful. They are just not comfortable, they are not at peace.

Love and fear are a duality. You have love and it's open and it's peaceful. It's the all, it's the expansion, being in presence in your life, in whatever way that is or whatever moment it is. It's opposite would then be fear.

Fear is what contracts everything. It's what makes things small. If you think about it, everything shrinks in a state of fear. Your life expands in proportion to your state of presence and love. It takes time to evolve into the knowing of the broader aspect of it so people are going through life, through the school of life. Unless you become conscious, then you are not really going to know. That's how I would look at it and describe knowing it now. If I had known what I know now many years ago, I wouldn't have suffered from a lot of anxiety and fear in my everyday life for so many years.

I look at the past, describing a journey in my life, just a story I'm telling that I have healed from that does not still wound me.

I know that so many people that are autistic go through a lot of anxiety and they are in fear a lot. That's because there's so much sensory overload, I can describe it like taking the plastic off of a plug and Al the wires are hanging out, akin to the nervous system overload, no shield. There's more unsettledness etc. and it's more difficult to handle everything when you have so many things happening at one time.

Going into primary at age 4, I was full of fear. I didn't know what I was facing into. I guess it's the fear of the unknown as well. I had no idea what was happening but I remember going in on the first day, and really being terrified. The teacher found someone to look after me for the day. I was so full of fear as a young child. But it was around the school. The fear was within me. Home was a quiet area and the middle of no where. I had not interacted with very many other people. Then suddenly, you are surrounded by all these people, a new teacher and new pupils.

I still feel that any child going to school would experience a certain amount of fear but I do feel that people that are on the spectrum experience it to a higher degree because of the overload and because we feel so much going on and even trying to be present generally is a struggle at times.

Using awareness as a grounding tool started at a very young age. I used to be outside most of the time growing up because I was in the countryside and absolutely grounded from doing what brings me into the moment.

This anxiety was always present in me, more of an underlying anxiety. I think a lot of people go through this underlying fear, like it's present all the time but they are not aware of it unless it becomes suddenly triggered and it becomes a heightened in the nervous system where it is hard to settle it. Some people may require treatment to settle it, whether it be medical intervention, or meditation, yoga, exercise, walking, running. Whatever works.

It pushed me as a younger person to achieve more but that was unhealthy and I was living on adrenaline at times. I don't see that as a positive now. I see and feel that there can be healthy competitions and healthy achievements.

There can be OCD perfection in that kind of thing which can really go over the top and make people quite sick, unwell and anxious.

Moving into secondary school was a different ball game altogether. A lot of fears came to the surface. I remember we were told what to anticipate. We were going into huge classes with a lot of people, a couple of hundred people and being seated in smaller groups. I remember quite vividly because of the stress. I spent a few months getting ready to go in there and wondering what this was going to be like as people were telling me about it.

I do remember having huge anxiety going in there. I had huge stress and pressure to perform and keep up with everything. Then you have to contend with not just one classroom. You have lots of extra different classes and moving out of classes every 40 minutes to go into the next.

I recall feeling a lot of stress and pressure. During the third year of secondary school, I experienced a type of breakdown. I had no idea that I was autistic. I didn't know why I was in fear, I didn't know why I was anxious, I didn''t know why I was finding it so hard everyday. I struggled.

Looking back now, I see it clearly. I see how the spiral happened. It was tumultuous. I remember the first the first time I came to realise that something is not right with this kind of thing. I was relieved to come to a better understanding. People cope with different mechanisms. I ended up going for summer holidays and took some couple of months off. When you are burnt out, you have take some time off and come back again to start anew. That was the kind of cycle I had.

It was a normal thing in a way, doing it all and burning it out. When you don't know you are anxious and then you meltdown and fall off the cliff completely within yourself. I would do nothing for a month or two and try to relax and have some fun. Then I would come back to life. That was the way it was for me as a teenager.

As I got older, I became stronger. When I was in my final year, it became much easier and I had grown within myself.

Back then, I was smoking. We used to in different teenage groups to an area in the school, then start smoking. A lot of kids today are under a lot of pressure from social media, along with peer pressure. It's a never ending overload and I believe there needs to be more supports available. But there's definitely the need for people to know themselves and for people to get to know themselves. They need to know if they are anxious, where they are, what they need for themselves rather than being in the unknowing of it, I think that can be helpful.

I think if more people are taught this at a younger age, there will be more peaceful environment. It's just observing the body, observing the feelings in the body and being able to name the emotions. My transformation is completely different from what people might expect it to be because it has come from within. It has come from the heart.

The more you recognize that there's something in you that is not peaceful, the more it shifts and the more it becomes peaceful. Then there is trancendence and movement. Then you will realise that this is duality of the world. There are two sides of everything. There's nothing that doesn't have a duality. When you can see it without being in judgment of it all. You just sit back and observe it. It becomes much easier to become peaceful in yourself because you know you can't control other people, you can't control other situations. You can't control what's going to happen anytime. But you can control your own space, your response and reaction to this and that. When you realise that everything is out of control and not under control, then there's peaceful-ness that pervades this fear, things start to crack open.

I start with myself, I work on myself everyday. That's all I can do. I can't change what anyone else is going to do or how people are going to respond to me, how people are going to react, how people I'm going to meet in the day are going to be. It can challenging especially for autistic people because a lot of the time, there's a tendency to want to know what is going to happen next. But deeply it's rooted in fear because we feel more than the average person maybe. There's more heightened sense of needing reassurance of some sort. It's a kind of a need.

I feel that people can still move through it no matter who the person is and no matter where you are at. We can still move through it and recognize that this doesn't have to be the journey. It can be changed. We can actually rise above it and and not let it overcome us. That's it. I have evolved over the years. The way I look and seek to live my life now is in my own truth and light, just being true to who I am.

I prefer to talk about what works than what doesn't work because there's no point feeding into energy that is not open, loving or present.

Ultimately, I feel there's a need for people to be taught how to know their own emotions more, how to learn from other people. I had to learn from other people. I was guided. It's up to the person to take the reins. You can just guide them and see where it takes them. A lot of change can come when we know ourselves more. Life is a journey for everyone. It's not black and white. When we choose love, it's easier. Choose Love and let go of the rest.

CHAPTER EIGHT

AUTISM AND ALCOHOL

I want to talk about my own experience as it's the only experience valid to me 100%. I would like to speak about Autism and Alcohol. I would like to give a little background around the Autism diagnosis I have had. So basically, I was 35 when I was diagnosed as an autistic woman and had lived I should say and fumbled through life up until then. Then, it came to a point where there was no option really but to figure out what was going on because there was always a hole, there was always a gap, there was always something missing. It changed my life, the diagnosis. I really feel it opened up my life in some ways that wouldn't have been possible if I hadn't known.

In April 2014, I was assessed. I already knew myself beforehand that I was autistic. I only needed confirmation at that point. I just wanted someone to tell me what I already knew. I remember going for the assessment down in Cork, sitting, and knowing, while waiting for my assessment. I think I should say for females, the assessment criteria is not really what it could be and I'm sure it will improve with time. There were not many people at the time offering assessment.

I was formally diagnosed with Asperger Syndrome. So basically, from that i had a huge healing. There was a huge healing process going through me because I had lived my whole life in the unknowing of this, fumbling and tumbling through life, finding things quite difficult.

So I went off, trying to get my hands on all the information I could get around women and Autism. I remember attending an event at UCC at that time, there were some speakers talking about Autism at this event. I was in the audience, just watching them. I remember sitting there, just putting my hand up. I needed to speak out about a few things and afterwards, I was asked to do an interview. I said 'Oh yes, great' and afterwards, I said to myself, "God, do I really want to do this?" But I ended up going ahead with my first feeling which was of course to go ahead and do it.

But it was a tough process. I did the interview and the article was published in the Irish Times newspaper in July 2014. I was at work at the time and I remember my whole life and my whole world really did change on that day in a lot of ways. It changed obviously within work because I had to make a disclosure. I made a full disclosure at my workplace and then I went out to the world. That's just a quick background of my diagnosis, my assessment, my coming out. Then, I did a few radio interviews after that and things settled down again. But I had a healing to go through my whole life up to that point.

Before I knew I was autistic, I was living a normal life per say. I started drinking in my teenage years. Looking at the alcohol side, I really didn't know I was anxious. I think it's a subconscious thing that there's anxiety. I wasn't aware of it. So I feel I wasn't really aware of why I was drinking at the time. As a teenager, you know what most teenagers do, we were drinking, smoking, having a great time, so we thought. It went on like that. I remember leaving school and moving on into the adult world. Still you're going out. I went out a lot and enjoyed being out. I was a social person. It was just a part of my life. It wasn't something that I thought about. What we did, myself, my friends and others, we went out. We had a good time and we had a few drinks. I think it did give confidence and it did kill the anxiety without me realising it, it was sedative.

Moving on from that, I was 19 years of age and I started travelling around with a 2 piece band. So I would like to say again that I was a very social person at night. In the day if I wasn't working, then I would take downtime, sleep. I wouldn't be a regular person, but there might be a lot people who might not be able to do that. But for me, it was an easy thing to do. I enjoyed singing. I enjoyed being out and we travelled around. So basically, that entailed four nights a week, drinking and getting free drink and just being able to have that at your disposal and subconsciously not really knowing the situation was out of control. This continued, I suppose looking at life now, it continued unconsciously. We continued travelling around with the band for eight years. In that time, I also had my children. I was with my partner at the time, eight years travelling with the band to gigs and drinking four or maybe five times a week and in all ways, I still functioned, working in daytime, studying in college and looking after my children outside of that. But knowing what I know now, obviously that was devastating in some ways to my life and in some ways, I still functioned.

Like I said, the cycle continued and I always functioned. But I had people come into my life inadvertently. One lady was a counsellor. She came into my life when I was 19.. Without her, probably I wouldn't have survived that period of time. I remember her sitting and having a conversation with me. I used to go to her a lot. I used to have an informal counselling session about life, about how things were. I remember her bringing up the alcohol and saying to me, 'You know you could die if you keep drinking'. But at that same time, I was a functioning person so I couldn't fully relate to what she was saying or the way she was talking because I didn't see anything wrong with the way life was. But then, I had no insight at the time. So the only way I can explain it is not having enough insight to see what other people could see. That has obviously changed after many years of work.

So the situation was what it was. I didn't know that I was autistic. I didn't know why there was no "shut off" button where you say, "Gosh, you need to stop this now.". That wasn't there. I feel that was the reason why I had no feeling of too much, no shut off point.

I always had a passive death wish, also at times a conscious death wish but I didn't quite know why.

But I did drink less in the next few years and what the counsellor said did trigger some slow changes in me where I became a little more aware overtime and she remained in my life until age 27 and on off after that. She was an angel and the first of 5 to 6 more to follow.

At the age of 27, I decided to explore the healing path firstly through Reiki healing, learning how to channel my inner healing, inner knowing and I learned how to meditate. That was the game changer. So I really think that without that I still wouldn't know myself if it took a long time. So the meditation and learning had to do that. It took a long time, a long time because my brain was so erratic and I really had no concentration span. There was no shift, like I used to sit down to try to meditate and get back up and leave the room. I couldn't do it. It was impossible to me for a while. It took years to make myself settle down and be able to do it.

But while I was learning it, I was also learning other modalities of healing. I was opening up more into self awareness. Then in my thirties, I was teaching meditation groups, giving readings and bringing people into their own self healing journeys. That took a long time, it was 8 years on from where I started out with healing. I'm bringing up alcohol and cigarettes because I used to smoke. I smoked for twenty years and again that was anxiety in different situations I found myself.

I feel that there are many men and women like me. I feel that most people like me are considered to be very high functioning, but we all struggle and our levels largely depend on situations or environments that we are in. It is not accurate to say we are high functioning across the board or that it doesn't change if we meltdown or are under a lot of stress. People can really struggle with anxiety and depression without knowing where the black hole is, the emotional pain. Why can't I feel that? What is that in me that I can't feel? So I'm drinking, I'm smoking on this. I do feel that there are probably many people who don't have the awareness, like I didn't have the awareness of why they do it, of what is behind it. There's a coping mechanism and there can be functioning people but still addicted to alcohol, etc. I just happened to be addicted to alcohol and cigarettes.

So I feel telling the story at times that it might release the old. It's really good. It's also good expression. It's a good way of communicating. It's good to open up to that, it's compartmentalized and I think being autistic, at times I can really compartmentalize different aspects of life and put them away, take them out some other time. I can do that quite easily, in some ways it can be very good and in some ways, it can be damaging. It can mean emotional suppression and not dealing with the emotional aspects of situations. So I think alcohol and cigarettes suppressed all the pain, all this unknowing of myself, this unsurety of self, and some sabotaging behaviour and all the rest of it. It's all part of that time and life was just into one jumble and you're just on automatic pilot, you're very unconscious. To go through that and then come out the other side of it and many years later feel extremely aware, self aware and conscious, it's a real miracle actually. It's really powerful and empowering to look at what is possible and I would say that is also possible for other people in their lives. People came into my life and helped me. I didn't even know I needed help. But there are so many people that need that belief in them. If people didn't believe in me, I would never have succeeded in doing what I have done, learning what I have learned, and turning my life around and changing everything. It wouldn't have happened without people standing there with me and knowing that there's more in me, I could do more, and that I had the capability for more.

I feel there are a lot of people that need to be heard, a lot of people find it difficult to express it. I could talk a lot but still find it hard to express myself in some ways. It's very important to just try and move past that and put ourselves out there for the people who are struggling and who don't have hope, who are trapped in different addiction cycles.

There's this lack of understanding in the general public arena around Autism. But it's starting to change, looking at people who are starting to come out and speak.

There's a huge gap. There's a need to meet the needs of different individuals, there are so many people. Like you might just meet my need as one autistic person. There are so many people who are not like me but there might be some similarities. But they might not be like me at all. They might just need something completely different so we need different people to come and talk about it, share how it is for them.

We can't assume that everyone is the same as one person or everyone else like somebody you meet on the spectrum. We can't assume they have nothing to say if they don't speak. We can't assume anything. For me, I find it awakening everyday, looking at people that are now starting to come out now and speak. We are learning from each other. It''s very important that everyone gets heard even if their opinion is not the same as someone else's opinion, that's their truth. Everyone needs to be heard in their own way.

So I've learned a lot. I gave up smoking and drinking 7 years ago. I feel as such a sensitive person, it's made a huge difference. My life is completely different to what it was in the past. It will never be the same and it opens up more everyday, just feeling, feeling life, and allowing life. Whereas before, it was blocking out life. Everything was too much. Now, I have learned to open to life more and more.

I had many mentors, some fantastic people who I have learned from and without them, I wouldn't be where I am now, with everything. There have been very dark times in my life. Very dark times, between depression and anxiety and etcetera. And now, it's the complete opposite. It's complete 360 change. My life couldn't be better. Everyday, I am going through a process, everyday Meditation, Prayer, Mindfulness, changing the Neuropath in the brain, the Heart entrains the brain (Lady Emmanuella, twitter handle: @onhi.) I have a good life. Life is very good. I have very good support and but that doesn't mean there are no challenges everyday. We have to battle. It's important to see the positives and to work on that. I keep working towards that.

Well, if I was more aware of myself, I wouldn't have gone into a lot of different situations I ended up in perhaps.

Perhaps I would have been more aware of pitfalls and of people taking advantage of your innocence and your good nature and other things that came with it. Not everybody did that but as a young person and a young girl growing up, you do meet that. You do meet I suppose many different situations. If I look back now, all I can say is I am here, I survived and I am grateful. I have a good life. I have learned a lot about myself. I have learned a lot about people, about trying to relate with people. But attempting to create friendship and different relationships...it's a challenge. Yes, it's a challenge. Although everyday is a challenge, I feel that with this strength everyday and being able to speak out gives us strength. It gives us the power to lift other people out of the despair, help them out of the harshness of alcoholism and drug addiction.

There's light in all of us and if you can be somebody who can emit light, I think there's a lot of hope for the future, for people out there. So I really do feel it's important to keep speaking about us. That's part of how my brain works.

I'm very easy on myself now. I'm gentle with myself, with who I am. I don't beat myself up. I am absolutely accepting of how things are. How my life has been now. I went through the healing and came out the other side. I just feel that if people are more aware than blaming others, they'll be better.

We need to look at people individually. We shouldn't write people off because they have a label or because they might be different. Everyone is different. It doesn't matter who we are. Nobody's got to be the same as you anyway, whether you're classed to be on the spectrum or you are not. We all have our uniqueness. I just feel there's a real need for respect, there's a need for understanding around things generally. There's need for more open conversation and more forums where people can chat these things and really connect. I think that's very important. There's no point in us hiding away, not being able to come out for fear of backlash or whatever. I don't hold fear around that. I just feel that I am who I am. I don't need to be anyone else just to suit people. A lot of people are comfortable with that and that's ok. I'm quite content with who I am, that's all that matters to me.

But I feel a lot of people are not there. There needs to be more compassion, there needs to be more open heartedness, and also open mindedness around things. I believe a lot of people are struggling especially with covid at the time and with the impact it left in their lives. So many people are struggling. You don't have to be autistic to be struggling. There are people struggling with innumerable things. But it's time to be kind, and be more compassionate around things, and now more than ever. We can connect in whatever way we can and this is the amplification of truth. So much is coming to light and so much is being revealed. This is really a good time to be living in.

CHAPTER NINE

NEURODIVERSITY

Looking at empowerment, I would describe it from the angle of emotional intelligence. This is what I would have used in my own life in one way or the other and in meditative practices. Take for example somebody who cannot control their emotions, they find it difficult to regulate their emotions and to regulate their lives in turn. It's good to look at how that can be changed.

I was someone who could not regulate my emotions at one stage. For most of my life, I was managing, but only until I was overwhelmed and had meltdowns, either mentally, emotionally, or physically. I didn't know or understand how to regulate my emotions.

It came to a stage where as I got older, I wanted things to be different, I wanted to feel different, I wanted to feel relaxed and I wanted to feel peaceful inside. I didn't want to feel so anxious. My nervous system was heightened. For quite a long time, I used to suffer from a lot of panic attacks. My nervous system was heightened, panic attack after panic attack. It continued for a while and I really did break down completely 14 years ago, I had a complete breakdown because I was trying to do too much of everything all at once. It was a culmination of many things. My body just said, 'no, we are not doing this anymore', my emotional body, my mental body, my physical body, my spiritual self, a whole lot of me just went, 'no'. I spent a while unable to do anything and I had to build up from the beginning.

Even though I had started my healing journey, it was after that I catapulted into the journey I am on now, the journey that has continued into awakening and into more knowing of self, life and God. That spurred me on to go deeper, to try to figure out who am I, what am I and why am I here.

I did not want to be in the world and that's where the breaking point comes for people when it becomes hard to be in the world that we feel is not geared towards us. I did hit that point quite a few times where I just didn't want to be here. I kept asking myself, what is this all about? What am I supposed to do? How can I do things better? Why is so difficult and challenging for me?

So it was all these things that led to deeper spiritual practice for me, meeting people along the path, my particular path. It's not meant for everybody. These people helped me to see more of myself and to uncover ways of figuring things out. So I was introduced to emotional intelligence at the seminar I attended. Credit for the seminar and for Love, Light and Truth goes to Lady Emmanuella, twitter handle: @onhi. It was here my life was uplifted.

Emotional intelligence is the ability to understand, use and manage your own emotions in positive ways to relieve stress, communicate effectively, empathize with others, overcome challenges and defuse conflict. When you look at all that in a nutshell, on paper it looks easy but it's not. It's a challenge. It's a challenge to even figure out what that means when you are actually saying to yourself, What am I supposed to do? How does that come about? I had to experience the coming about of it within myself. I didn't understand just reading it. You could say you could understand this but how do you bring it into your life? It's clearly a different thing.

Basically, if you are looking to try and manage your own emotions in a positive way, then you have to realise that your emotions are out of control. You have to realise that there's an issue. I was in the world, in work, functioning independently and attempting to do all this. Often people don't realise they have an issue in the first place with controlling their emotions.

Some people are self aware and some are not yet self aware. Some time back, I wouldn't have said to myself that I had an issue with my emotions or how I processed them. That wasn't something I thought. But I didn't have the insight to see that. So people have to first of all realise that there might be something that needs to be changed. Maybe I need to look at myself instead of looking at everyone else and always projecting out into the society. 'It's their fault. I can't do this. I have all these ideas to change the world but it's their fault.' So we have to turn it back in on ourselves and ask what we can do then to be out in the world the way they are, do what they do on the same level. What do I need to do because they can't do it for me. One thing is that nobody came in and did it for me.

I got pointers, I had a lot of mentors. I had a lot of people who knew I would figure it out. I figured it out. So it was me who had to do the work. And everyday I had to do the work. It didn't stop after a month. This is going on for years and everyday I have to do the work because I'm still in the world that isn't particularly geared for me in so many ways. But I'm learning. I have learned a lot to adapt in ways I can and I have had things adapt to me where necessary. So you know you are willing to go and meet it half way as well. That's important.

With emotional intelligence, you are relieving stress. That's obvious. If our bodies and nervous systems are very heightened and sensory overloaded, then we must find ways that suit us as individuals to relieve our stress. I relieve my stress in whatever way I need to. I will meditate, I will sit down and read and be in silence. I could go to nature, the beach, whatever works. But it's figuring it out first of all that's most important. You can make a list of what works for you then work from there.

Communication of course is a huge one especially for autistic people. Sometimes I could be talking to somebody and I would be having a conversation, I might as well have been speaking in some other language because they take me up completely wrong and things can turn out in a way that you never anticipated.

It's quite challenging for us to try to communicate what we want and get it out in a way that somebody would take a long enough to listen and to understand it from what you are trying to say rather than what they are assuming. This can happen in all relationships especially with autistic people and even in our own community as well. People can misunderstand each other. That's not a myth.

Although it's challenging, we just keep working it out, accepting that this is going to be a bit of a challenge. But if we communicate and try and communicate effectively then we got to keep doing it. That's the way I get through things.

You just don't give up. You just go back to the drawing board again and you try a new approach. We need to look deeper and find out what we need to improve and how to do that.

Empathy. I do feel that a lot of autistic people are hugely empathetic. Obviously, there might be those that aren't. But i really know that everybody I met on the spectrum that is autistic is very empathetic. We feel so much. The emotions are so strong and we feel everything, situations, people, environments, rooms, everything.

Putting yourself in someone else's shoes is huge. So we practised sometimes like If you have a disagreement with somebody, what is it like for them? What are they feeling? How would I feel if I was in their shoes? We did a little bit of that in order not to be so self absorbed.

The tendency to be self absorbed is easy, it's easy to be selfish. It takes effort to change this. This needs to be looked at as well. We need to look at our behaviours, our own emotions and how they affect other people. It's important that we are aware, have the insight and we are capable of doing that. You can go into the world expecting acceptance but we must also do the work to meet that. You can't just sit down and do nothing and complain about everyone saying the society is awful.

When people are advocating which is fantastic, just remember that you want to be met at the level you are bringing so we've got to come to it from the heart. We have to come to it from a place where we genuinely want to meet the society and have the expectation that they want to meet us. We have got to rise up to that as well regardless of how we feel that people have treated us in the past. Not everybody will treat us badly. They just haven't learned how to do it and they just don't really know.

I think there's a lot of fear around who and what we are sometimes. When people get to know us, they realise we are not so different after all. We just have our own way of being and thinking.

Overcoming challenges is an everyday thing. We overcome challenges all the time. So defusing conflict like I said is about people meeting each other where they are both at, even if they don't agree, even if they have different opinions and still managing to come together, even live together or work together. This isn't just for autistic people. This is in general.

It's important to look at how we can make it better. How can we work together to make things better for others.

Self awareness for me is meditation. It won't be that for everyone. Meditation can happen in a lot of ways. You don't have to sit down and close your eyes to meditate. You can wash dishes and meditate and be very present in that moment. You could be driving and meditate by just being aware. Awareness of knowing oneself is sufficient.

A lot of my learning has come from a lot of spiritual teachers as well and I would be an advocate of The Power of Now and The Law of Attraction. It works. I'm living it. Through living it, we understand how it works. Then we start to realise that we create our lives all the time. So if you don't want to create something, then you don't need to do it, not think, not feel that, not put your energy into it. If you want to expand something, put your energy into it. It's fabulous. It's about taking responsibility for what we are creating ourselves, how that plays out in our lives, how that plays out in other people's lives, how that plays out in the whole collective environment. We start to realise that we are not powerless. I feel society needs to realise that we as autistic people have the potential to become extremely empowered. That's happening. As I said, there's a shift now. So that's going to be seen all over the world soon.

A realization of respect and understanding that we all have the power to create and work is important. Sometimes we can do it in different ways. We don't necessarily think in the same way or do it the same way, feel the same way about things. It's really about coming together, it's about whatever we are creating, what we desire to come about, what we expect to come about as a community.

So self regulation goes with self awareness. I'm so aware now that I allow myself the time to process things and I also allow other people the time to process. If I get a text message or an email, I often don't reply until the next day because I just haven't processed it.

Also, motivation is something that needs to come from within as well. People can motivate you but they can't do it for you, they can't come and make you get up in the morning. That's not empowerment, that's control. That's running someone's life. That's making them into something that they are not, trying to control the situation or how their lives should be lived. You have people who do that. There are a lot of autistic people who suffer because of that. There are people who come in, thinking they know what's best for them and decide how their lives should be. Where's the autonomy in that? Where's the empowerment in that? So that's not it. People need to be allowed to find their own space to motivate themselves. All they need is a little guide. But they need the space to figure it out, they need the space to be able to live in whatever that they wish to live. As far as they are not harming themselves or others, people are entitled to live in the way they want to live that is good for them.

I'm very lucky in the work that I do. Over the past few years, my work has become stronger and stronger, the desire to sit with people who are in distress. That's what I do predominantly. When I get to work, as an agency worker, I usually work on a one to one speciality. It depends. If I'm with someone who is usually in deep stress, that's a huge honour and it's a huge gift to be allowed to sit with people in that state. I see it a lot of the time as a social crisis for them and an awakening. There are times that I see that there's a huge need for a change in the way that this is done within the services, in the way that these people are responded to. I work with a lot of people. I would say that about 30 percent of the people I work with are autistic and you have other mental illnesses covering the rest but you meet people. They fall into similar spectrum but you meet people who for the most part are extremely distressed and often suicidal. That's my role. I feel that people should be given the space in their lives in order to maybe not reach that point where they are so down, where before they reach that point, they would receive help through the proper channel that would allow for emotional intelligence to arise. Courses should be run in this way and more holistically.

I'm not a staunch advocate for anything in particular. I think everything has its place and everything can work. It's not that I just want to be holistic but I feel it needs to be looked at that half of these people could probably have been prevented from getting to this point. I know there could be prevention around it.

So it's very important that people are respected as people in their own right, their right to live their own lives in the way they want even if people think that's not okay but it's okay. It's okay for people to be themselves.

The other thing is social skills in general. There's a need for autistic people to learn certain social skills because without that, life would be more stressful. I use myself as an autistic person as an example. It's not about fitting in that regard, it's about being able to go out comfortably and not feel stressed and to figure out there are certain places where we will be and we will need not to fit in or blend in but to be a part of it, to try and share it with other people. In that case, it's good to meet people half way and not to just want it all our way.

When we go somewhere, we must be willing to give and take with others in different situations. I can't go into my work and decide that I'm not going to do it the way they do it. I can't do that. I will work 100% professionally with them but I will also bring myself into that work. I won't disregard the work they are doing and that I'm trained to do. I will add the flavour of the holistic side through who I am, through my presence.

All these things have worked for me and continues to work for me. I'm using it all the time. It's an everyday thing. It hasn't changed. I don't stop trying to improve. I now have a strong knowing of myself, who I am, what I want, what I don't want, what I like, what I don't like, what works for me, what doesn't work for me. I have learned all of that just overtime, from wanting to and following the inner guidance as well as the meditation that I do. These tools have got me to where I am today. You are welcome to follow my Facebook pages, all of these things have helped me to know that I'm in my truth and when I go about my day, I feel that I'm in my truth. What I'm doing is coming from a genuine place without any kind of ulterior motives. That's a nice feeling. It's very important to be self aware, to be present. So find what it is for you.

Nobody can give you empowerment. Nobody can come and say I will empower you now. They can help you and point you in the direction. It has to come from inside, you have to have the desire to rise up. When we hit the bottom, where I have been, we have to make a choice then. What do I want? Do I want to be like this forever? Do I want things to change? Then the empowerment starts to unfold. You have to accept that it's not an easy journey but you have to make it in order to be in that comfortable place in your life. It was not an easy choice but I made it. I am happy I made the choice.

CHAPTER TEN

THE POWER OF LOVE IN ACTION

I feel that when Love is put into action it is here that it multiplies, when people are giving freely with no expectation of a return.

Sometimes weve got to sit and ask ourselves. What is my agenda here ? What is my motive for doing what I am doing ? Am I doing this from the heart or for personal gain?

I've been drawn to different types of charity work over many years, because it makes me feel like I am contributing something. Not that I am an amazing person, but it gives me joy. Uplifting others in some way brings me joy. It gives me a sense of purpose outside of my everyday life and work. I have always felt the hand of God the strongest through me and in situations when I am doing this work.

I have met amazing people through this work and I would highly recommend it to anyone who feels that they need a purpose or that anything is lacking in their lives. It will empower you to realise that there are so many people suffering around us that need compassion, and love and help. In whatever way we can bring it to them.

I have been involved in various different settings and I've enjoyed each one thoroughly. I began with the soup run in Limerick city going back to 2010 with Novas Initiatives who do great work. From there i volunteered in a charity shop and in later years I went to Kolkata to volunteer in Shishu Bhavan which is an orphanage for children with disabilities, this place broke my heart open in a very deep way. The overwhelming sadness I felt in my heart for them all. 26 children in cots and on a mat for feeding times during the day. The first day I arrived a young girl was leaving her baby as she could not keep the child and was forced into that position in truth. The only real advantage here is that are many volunteers from different countries as it is so well known due to Mother Teresa and its very close proximity to the Mothethouse. Very much a learning, a lot of tears cried there and also experiencing a completely different culture. I do aim to go back in the right timing and see them again.

Following this I spent a brief time in Calais with a charity called Care4Calais where we were working in groups delivering supplies to the refugees that were there and chatting with them and hearing their stories. The group does amazing work and has worked in tough conditions, in freezing conditions, and solely on the donations that they receive. I also had the opportunity just for one day to travel to Brussels and to offer relief and clothing etc to the refugees that were there. It was wonderful to drive there and back in a matter of hours. Grateful for the experiences. All were pre covid time.

At the moment I feel I'm at a bit of a loose end as its been a while now since I have volunteered but I'm currently in Mallorca so I will again do so when the opportunity arises.

Please do check out the above charities and organisations if you are interested in doing similar. All the experiences have been amazing and really it takes me out of my own story and mind to focus more on the reality of the suffering that is around us.

We cannot set ourselves apart from this. All suffering is indeed our suffering as a whole. When one suffers we all suffer. Its important now in the times that we are in to answer that call when it arises within our hearts. To stand as the time is upon us to act. Not to sit back and merely wait on others to do so.

This begins with treating all life with love, respect and compassion. Also treating ourselves with the same love, respect and compassion that we give to others.

My wish is for unity for us all to realise that we are indeed one. Our hearts are one. Whether we are Autistic or not. All of life is interconnected and we are interdependent in truth. All is weaved into one. Time will change many things. We have an opportunity to very quickly try to change the trajectory for ourselves. We need to take it and do what we can where we are.

The time is NOW

EPILOGUE

We are all one. Whether we are Autistic or Neurotypical. In the heart it does not matter. If we are to look at eachother through the eyes of the heart then we will only see light and love. There will be no judgement of eachother in essence.

I ask you to look deep within your hearts and realise this connection to eachother. Before you judge or assume, sit and feel with your heart how challenging it is for each and every human being on the planet in one way or another. We all carry the weight of our own realities. We all have battles at times, challenges, losses, and gains.

Ultimately when we surrender our hearts to God and accept our path and purpose. Only good can come from this. Choose Love over fear. Choose Love over hate, Love over judgement, Peace over war. Becoming peaceful is the key to change in every moment. Choosing Peace and Love within our hearts.

Thank you for reading
Paula Nash

Facebook Page - My Autistic Heart
Facebook Page - Divine Heart and Soul Readings/Initiations/Soul Purpose Alignment
Twitter - @paulanash1
Email: Paulanash0@gmail.com

HEALING SERVICES OFFERED

Heart and Soul Readings - Reiki Initiations Level 1 Level 2 and Level 3 (Mastership)

Munay KI Initiations - Soul Purpose Alignment - Spiritual Healing and Direction

Indian Head Massage - Magnified Healing

Reiki Tummo - Seichem - Crystal Healing

Integrated Energy Therapy - Emotional Freedom Techniques - Yin Yoga Classes

Meditation Classes - Heart Healing

I have spent over 20 years in the development of the above practices and it is in surrender to God that i practice and offer services both confidentially and with high integrity, truth and non judgement.